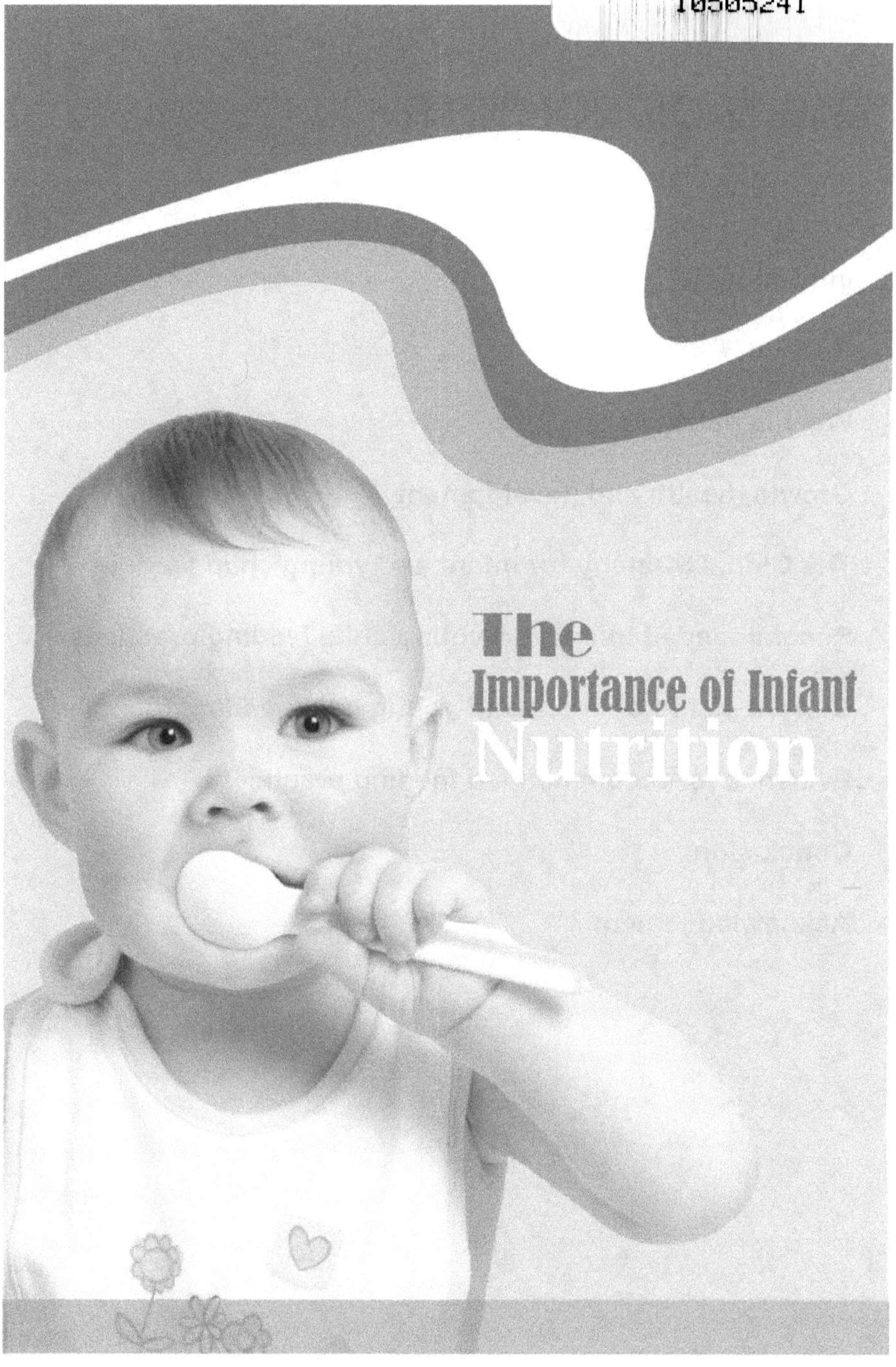

The
Importance of Infant
Nutrition

TABLE OF CONTENT

NTRODUCTION

For a baby, breast milk is best. It has all the necessary vitamins and minerals. Infant formulas are available for babies whose mothers are not able to or decide not to breastfeed. Infants are usually ready to eat solid foods at about 6 months of age.

Preface

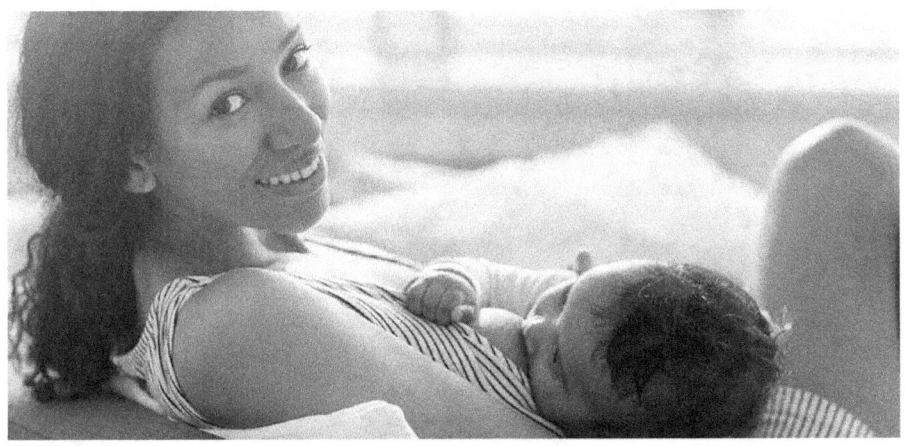

What is nutrition

Nutrition is the process of taking in food and converting it into energy and other vital nutrients required for life." Nutrients are the substances which provide energy and biomolecules necessary for carrying out the various body functions. All living organisms need nutrients for proper functioning and growth.

Good nutrition during the first 2 years of life is vital for healthy growth and development. Starting good nutrition practices early can help children develop healthy dietary patterns.

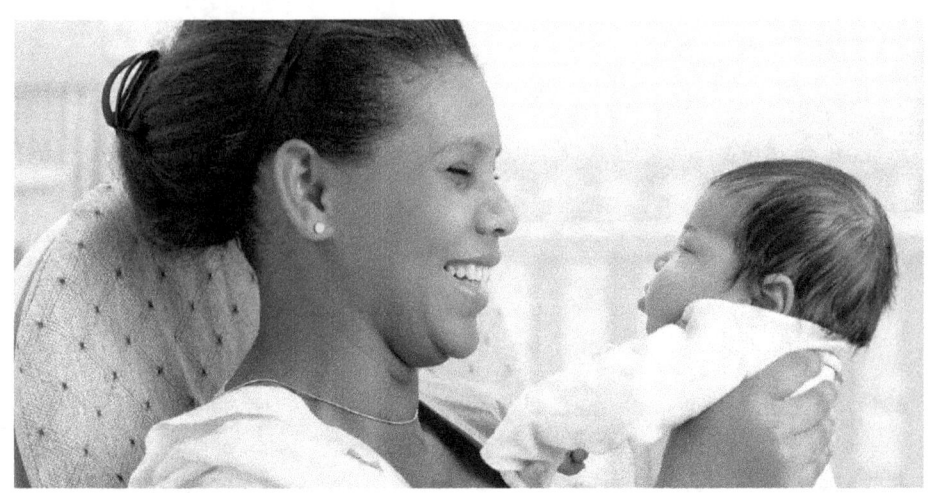

Growth, Health and Development

Adequate nutrition during infancy and early childhood is essential to ensure the growth, health, and development of children to their full potential. Poor nutrition increases the risk of illness, and is responsible, directly or indirectly, for one third of the estimated 9.5 million deaths that occurred in 2006 in children less than 5 years of age. Inappropriate nutrition can also lead to childhood obesity which is an increasing public health problem in many countries.

Early nutritional deficits are also linked to long-term impairment in growth and health. Malnutrition during the first 2 years of life causes stunting, leading to the adult being several centimeters shorter than his or her potential height. There is evidence that adults who were malnourished in early childhood have impaired intellectual performance. They may also have reduced capacity for physical work. If women were malnourished as children, their reproductive capacity is affected, their infants may have lower birth weight, and they have more complicated deliveries. When many children in a population are malnourished, it has implications for national development. The overall functional consequences of malnutrition are thus immense.

The first two years of life provide a critical window of opportunity for ensuring children's appropriate growth and development through optimal feeding. Based on evidence of the effectiveness of interventions, achievement of universal coverage of optimal breastfeeding could prevent 13% of deaths occurring in children less than 5 years of age globally, while appropriate complementary feeding practices would result in an additional 6% reduction in under-five mortality.

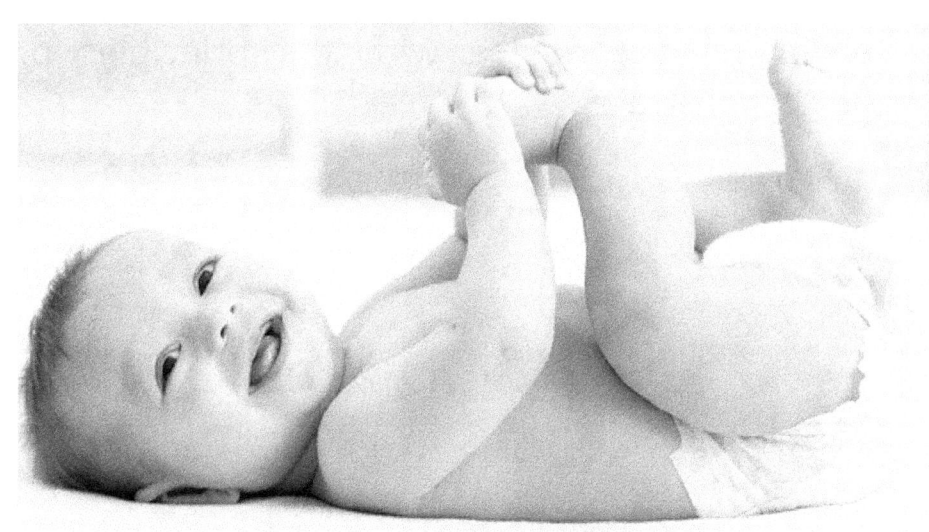

The Global Strategy for Infant and Young Child Feeding

In 2002, the World Health Organization and UNICEF adopted the Global Strategy for infant and young child feeding. The strategy was developed to revitalize world attention to the impact that feeding practices have on the nutritional status, growth and development, health, and survival of infants and young children. This Model Chapter summarizes essential knowledge that every health professional should have in order to carry out the crucial role of protecting, promoting and supporting appropriate infant and young child feeding in accordance with the principles of the Global Strategy.

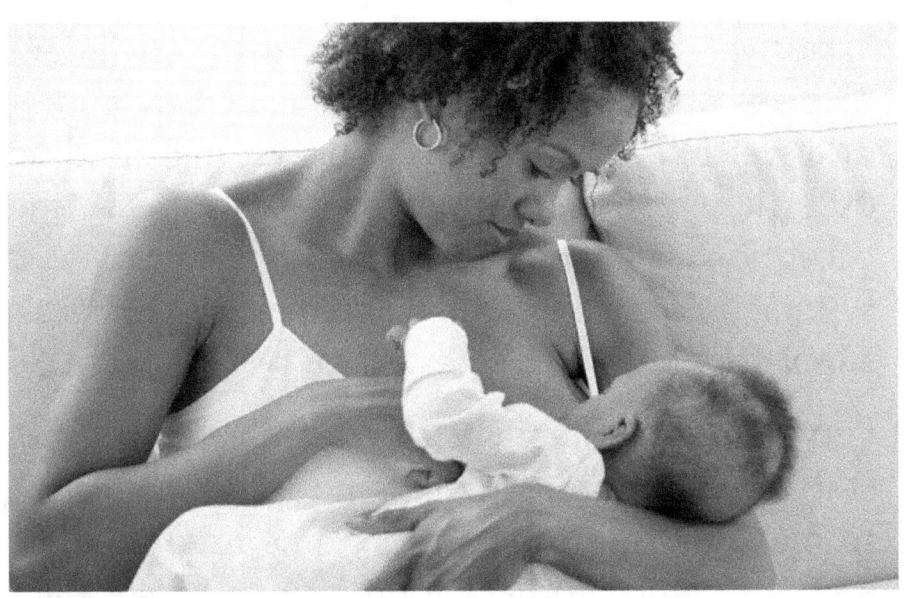

Recommended Infant and Young Child Feeding Practices

WHO and UNICEF's global recommendations for optimal infant feeding as set out in the *Global Strategy* are:

- exclusive breastfeeding for 6 months (180 days)

- nutritionally adequate and safe complementary feeding starting from the age of 6 months with continued breastfeeding up to 2 years of age or beyond.

Exclusive breastfeeding means that an infant receives only breast milk from his or her mother or a wet nurse, or expressed breast milk, and no other liquids or solids, not even water, with the exception of oral rehydration solution, drops or syrups consisting of vitamins, minerals supplements or medicines.

Complementary feeding is defined as the process starting when breast milk is no longer sufficient to meet the nutritional requirements of infants, and therefore other foods and liquids are needed, along with breast milk. The target range for complementary feeding is generally taken to be 6 to 23 months of age, even though breastfeeding may continue beyond two years.

These recommendations may be adapted according to the needs of infants and young children in exceptionally difficult circumstances, such as pre-term or low-birth-weight infants, severely malnourished children, and in emergency situations. Specific recommendations apply to infants born to HIV-infected mothers.

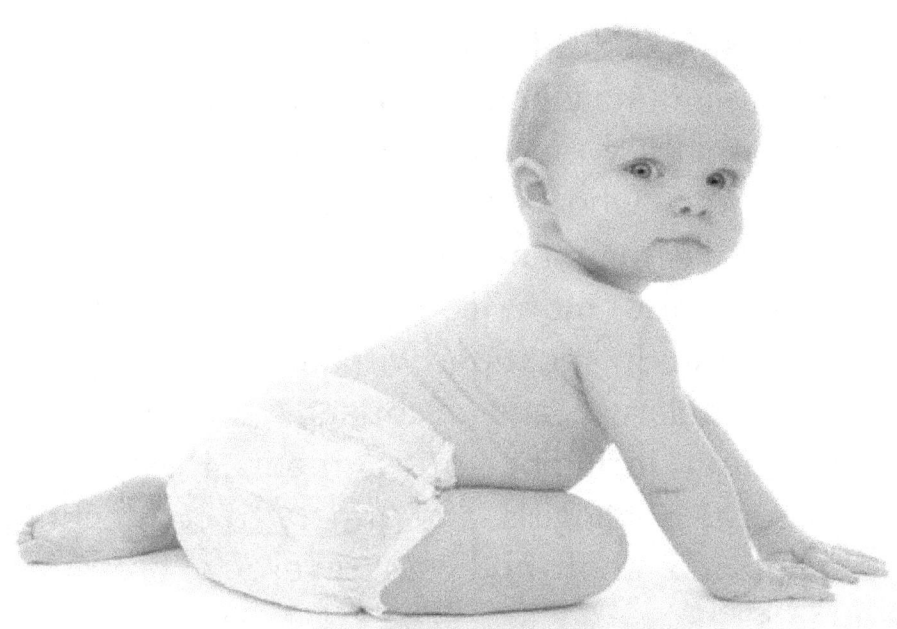

Evidence For Recommended Feeding Practices

Breastfeeding

Breastfeeding confers short-term and long-term benefits on both child and mother, including helping to protect children against a variety of acute and chronic disorders. The long-term disadvantages of not breastfeeding are increasingly recognized as important.

Reviews of studies from developing countries show that infants who are not breastfed are 6 to

10 times more likely to die in the first months of life than infants who are breastfed. Diarrhea and pneumonia are more common and more severe in children who are artificially fed, and are responsible for many of these deaths. Diarrhea illness is also more common in artificially-fed infants even in situations with adequate hygiene, as in Belarus and Scotland. Other acute infections, including otitis media, Hemophilus influenzae meningitis, and urinary tract infection, are less common and less severe in breastfed infants.

Artificially-fed children have an increased risk of long-term diseases with an immunological basis, including asthma and other atopic conditions, type 1 diabetes, celiac disease, ulcerative colitis and Crohn disease. Artificial feeding is also associated with a greater risk of childhood leukemia.

Several studies suggest that obesity in later childhood and adolescence is less common among breastfed children, and that there is a dose response effect, with a longer duration of breastfeeding associated with a lower risk. The effect may be less clear in populations were some children are undernourished. A growing body of evidence links artificial feeding with risks to cardiovascular health, including increased blood pressure, altered blood cholesterol levels and atherosclerosis in later adulthood.

Regarding intelligence, a meta-analysis of 20 studies showed scores of cognitive functions on average 3.2 points higher among children who were breastfed compared with those who were formula fed. The difference was greater (by 5.18 points) among those children who were born with low birth weight. Increased duration of breastfeeding has been associated with greater intelligence in late childhood and adulthood, which may affect the individual's ability to contribute to society.

For the mother, breastfeeding also has both short- and long-term benefits. The risk of postpartum hemorrhage may be reduced by breastfeeding immediately after delivery, and there is increasing evidence that the risk of breast and ovarian cancer is less among women who breastfed.

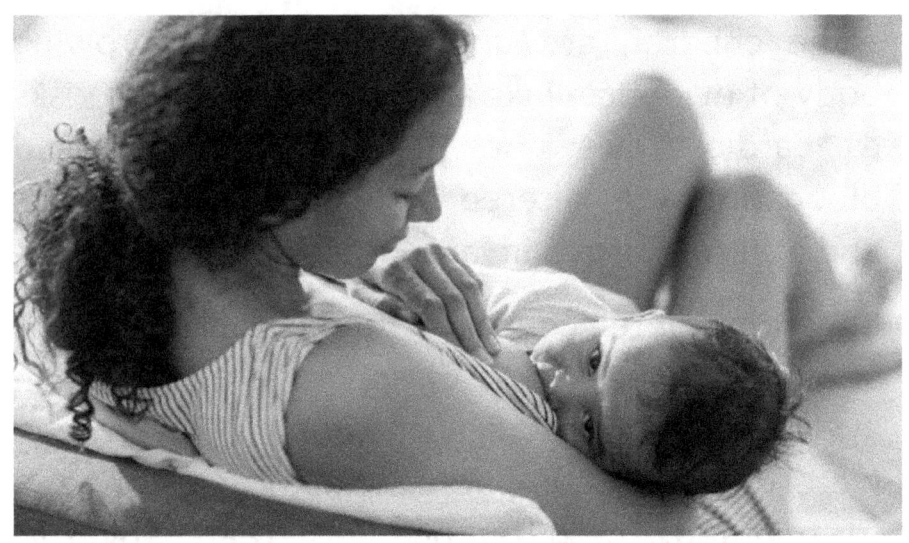

Breastfeeding for 6 months

The advantages of exclusive breastfeeding compared to partial breastfeeding were recognized in 1984, when a review of available studies found that the risk of death from diarrhea of partially breastfed infants 0–6 months of age was 8.6 times the risk for exclusively breastfed children. For those who received no breast milk the risk was 25 times that of those who were exclusively breastfed. A study in Brazil in 1987 found that compared with exclusive breastfeeding, partial breastfeeding was associated with 4.2 times the risk of death, while no breastfeeding had 14.2 times the risk. More recently, a study in Dhaka, Bangladesh found that deaths from diarrhea and pneumonia could be reduced by one third if infants were exclusively instead of partially breastfed for the first 4 months of life. Exclusive breastfeeding for 6 months has been found to reduce the risk of diarrhea and respiratory illness compared with exclusive breastfeeding for 3 and 4 months respectively.

If the breastfeeding technique is satisfactory, exclusive breastfeeding for the first 6 months of life meets the energy and nutrient needs of the vast majority of infants. No other foods or fluids are necessary. Several studies have shown that healthy infants do not need additional water during the first 6 months if they are exclusively breastfed, even in a hot climate. Breast milk itself is 88% water, and is enough to satisfy a baby's thirst. Extra fluids displace breast milk, and do not increase overall intake. However, water and teas are commonly given to infants, often starting in the first week of life. This practice has been associated with a two-fold increased risk of diarrhea.

For the mother, exclusive breastfeeding can delay the return of fertility, and accelerate recovery of pre-pregnancy weight. Mothers who breastfeed exclusively and frequently have less than a 2% risk of becoming pregnant in the first 6 months postpartum, provided that they still have amenorrhea.

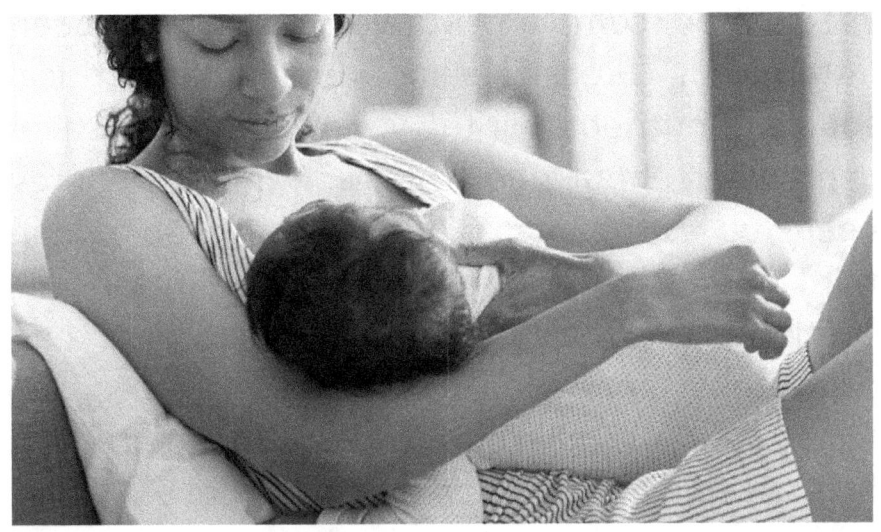

Complementary feeding from 6 months

From the age of 6 months, an infant's need for energy and nutrients starts to exceed what is provided by breast milk, and complementary feeding becomes necessary to fill the energy and nutrient gap. If complementary foods are not introduced at this age or if they are given inappropriately, an infant's growth may falter. In many countries, the period of complementary feeding from 6–23 months is the time of peak incidence of growth faltering, micronutrient deficiencies and infectious illnesses.

Even after complementary foods have been introduced, breastfeeding remains a critical source of nutrients for the young infant and child. It provides about one half of an infant's energy needs up to the age of one year, and up to one third during the second year of life. Breast milk continues to supply higher quality nutrients than complementary foods, and also protective factors. It is therefore recommended that breastfeeding on demand continues with adequate complementary feeding up to 2 years or beyond.

Complementary foods need to be nutritionally-adequate, safe, and appropriately fed in order to meet the young child's energy and nutrient needs. However, complementary feeding is often fraught with problems, with foods being too dilute, not fed often enough or in too small amounts, or replacing breast milk while being of an inferior quality. Both food and feeding practices influence the quality of complementary feeding, and mothers and families need support to practice good complementary feeding.

CONCLUSION

Correct feeding in the first three years of life is particularly important due to its role in lowering morbidity and mortality, reducing the risk of chronic disease throughout their life span, and promoting regular mental and physical development.

Infants should be breastfed or formula fed exclusively for the first six months of life. Infants should not consume solid foods prior to six months because solid foods do not contain the right nutrient mix that infants need. Also, eating solids may mean drinking less human milk or formula.

For a baby, breast milk is best. It has all the necessary vitamins and minerals. Infant formulas are available for babies whose mothers are not able to or decide not to breastfeed. Infants are usually ready to eat solid foods at about 6 months of age.

Nutrition is the process of consuming, absorbing,

and using nutrients needed by the body for growth, development, and maintenance of life. To receive adequate, appropriate nutrition, people need to consume a healthy diet, which consists of a variety of nutrients—the substances in foods that nourish the body.

Some toddlers have nutritional problems that can have immediate and long-term effects on their health, growth and development. Food allergies, iron deficiency, tooth decay and constipation are common in the early years.

One thing you don't want to give your baby during the first 12 months is whole cow's milk. It doesn't have enough iron, vitamin E, and essential fatty acids for your baby. Also, it contains too much protein, sodium, and potassium for your child's body to absorb and can cause harm. Wait to introduce cow's milk until your baby is 1 year old.

You also don't want to give your baby soy milk or homemade formula. These substitutes may not have the balance of nutrition baby needs right now.

ACKNOWLEDGEMENT

I would like to thank the God for the inspiration given to me to embark on this book journey and the success of the book, I also thank WHO and UNICEF, for there research material, also everybody that participated towards the success of this book.